Surviving Breast Cancer

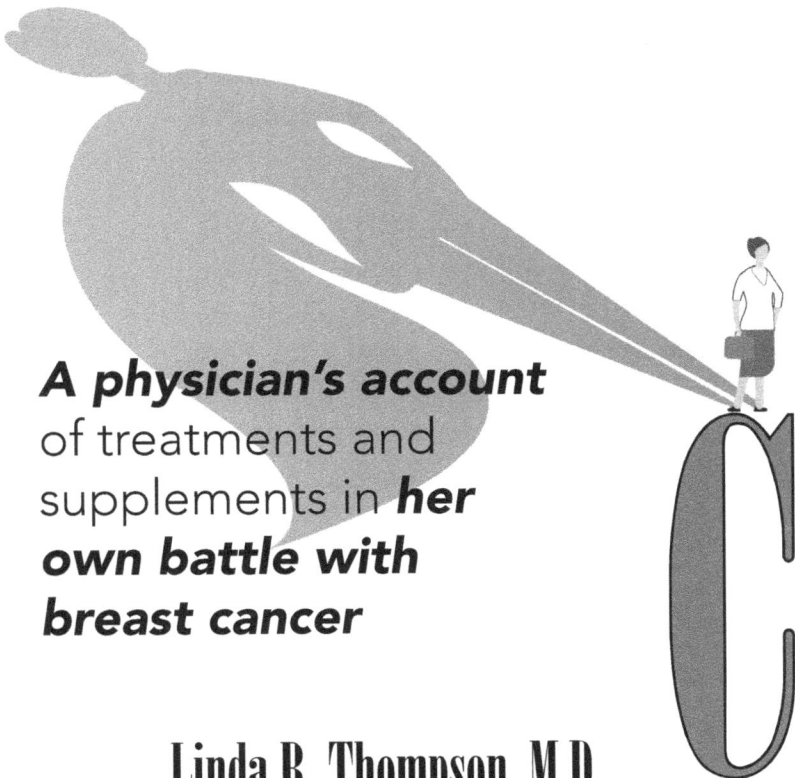

A physician's account of treatments and supplements in **her own battle with breast cancer**

Linda R. Thompson, M.D.

Published by Vision Run Publishing

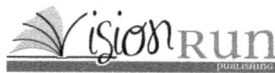

Dedicated to my exceptional

treatment team

Surviving Breast Cancer

CONTENTS

Disclaimer: Although the author and publisher have made every effort to ensure the information in this book was correct at press time, the author and publisher do not assume and hereby disclaim any liability to any party for any loss, damage, or disruption caused by errors or omissions, whether such errors or omissions result from negligence, accident, or any other cause. This is the author's personal story and not intended to prescribe, diagnose, or treat any illness or disease.

INTRODUCTION

In January of 2007 I was diagnosed with breast cancer. As a practicing physician and psychiatrist I had the advantage of knowing how to make medical decisions regarding treatments for cancer, and I also realized that most patients who have to deal with a diagnosis of cancer do not have a medical background. They are usually very anxious and willing to accept the doctor's recommendations for treatment. In most instances they receive good care because there are a lot of evidenced-based guidelines for the most common cancers and many treatments are standardized. However, there will always be individual patients whose cancer is either a very rare type or who have severe reactions to the standard treatments, necessitating the development of a more individualized treatment plan.

My purpose in writing this book is to provide information about the treatments for my breast cancer and the issues I had to make decisions about that were outside the usual guidelines. It is my hope that this information will be of benefit to other women with breast cancer, so they will be able to ask questions of their treating physicians regarding side effects of medications and/or other complications that may occur during the course of their treatment. Since I have been treated for breast cancer, as well as knowing something about the older cancer treatments from my medical education, I believe that I am uniquely qualified to provide some patient-centered information that addresses the issues of standard treatments, troubleshooting problems that occur in the course of treatment, some alternative treatments that have worked for me and some lifestyle changes that can optimize your health in general.

As for my professional credentials, I have been a practicing physician since graduating medical school at the University of Virginia School of Medicine in 1966. I did a rotating internship at the State University of Iowa Hospital in Iowa City, Iowa in 1966-1967, and my residency in psychiatry at the University of Virginia Hospital in 1967-1971. Following my residency, I was a staff psychiatrist at the Northern Virginia Mental Health Institute in Fairfax, Virginia for six months before going into a full-time private practice.

For 13 years, I practiced in the Washington DC area, doing primarily psychoanalytically-oriented psychotherapy. I was also enrolled as a candidate at the Washington Psychoanalytic Institute for psychoanalytic training. I completed that training in 1983. By then it was clear that insurance would no longer cover psychoanalytic treatment under the major medical supplement to many federal health insurance plans and the option of continuing a full-time psychoanalytic practice was no longer a viable option.

With an adjustment in the focus of my practice, I moved to the Tri-Cities area of northeast Tennessee and southwest Virginia in 1984 and established a general psychiatry practice. My work consisted of a part time private psychotherapy practice in combination with a consulting practice associated with regional mental health centers, where I provided psychiatric services for their clients. I also did psychiatric evaluations at some of the local community hospitals, seeing patients who were being treated for medical or surgical illnesses, but who also needed psychiatric interventions and/or evaluations. This gave me ongoing contact with some patients who were being treated for cancer, and enabled me to see the changes and improvements for various cancers during that time. I continued the consulting practice through August 2014.

As an observer of the changes in medical and psychiatric practices over the past 45 years, I have seen the shift in emphasis from patient-centered treatments to disease-specific treatments. This has been largely driven by insurance requirements and advances in available technologies and medications. In quite a few instances, the physicians do not listen to the patient's account of their symptoms and the responses and/or their problems with their treatments. Treatment decisions are made based on the evidence-based guidelines, which will not always be appropriate for a significant minority of their patients.

I have kept this book as brief as possible because I can remember that I did not want to read a lot of detailed information about my own cancer. My focus at that time was to just concentrate on getting through the treatments as best I could. That was one of the reasons why I chose to remain in my home community for the treatments. I also had personal knowledge about the doctors on my treatment team and I could comfortably trust their clinical recommendations.

In this book I have focused on the treatments, the unforeseen complications and my coping strategies during and after the treatments. I would also recommend obtaining a copy of Dr. David Derry's book Breast Cancer and Iodine that has been very helpful to me in thinking through the issues of long-term prevention of recurrence of my own cancer.

CHAPTER 1

Symptoms and Diagnosis

Having recently started a new diet over the Christmas holidays, I was feeling better generally going into the new year. I had gradually lost down to 183 pounds, counting the 15 pounds I had lost on the new diet. It wasn't a major change in what I was eating — just doing more salads with very simple dressings, like fresh squeezed lemon juice over greens and fruit. I was also drinking fruit smoothies daily. Sipping them throughout the workday in place of a regular lunch was working well for me. I had not yet discovered green smoothies, which are now part of my daily routine. At that time, I was only working 4 days a week and had more time to work out the new diet.

Then, one night in January 2007, I noticed some spots of blood on my bra, on the left side. I knew that cancer was the most likely cause. I did a breast exam but as usual, with my fibrocystic disease, I could feel more lumps than I could keep track of, and none of them felt that unusual. I have always found it impossible to effectively monitor my breasts for masses because of the cysts that have been there since my early teens.

There was no additional blood for about a week and then there was a larger spot of blood in my bra and a small amount of blood on the nipple. I called my gynecologist, Dr. Wendy Strawbridge, who is also a good friend, and she arranged an appointment for the next day. She also arranged for a mammogram to be done within a couple of days.

We talked about treatment options at that first appointment. Knowing it would be a long process, I did not want to travel out of my home area for the treatments. I had been working on the Med-Psych unit at the Bristol Regional Medical Center for several years from 1999 to 2003 and was familiar with most of the clinical staff there. I knew that I wanted Dr. Sue Prill to be my oncologist should I ever need that. I let Dr. Strawbridge know that that decision was already made. I was familiar with Dr. Prill's compassionate care of her patients. Overall her patients seemed to have fewer complications with their chemotherapy. And, when I first saw her as a patient, she told me straight off, no matter what other side effects I might have with the chemo, that I would definitely lose my hair. This presented a minor wardrobe delimma in that I rarely wear anything in the way of hats or scarves. In fact, I don't really like anything on my head. But I had to suck it up and wear a wig for eight or nine months; it was a great relief when I could finally get rid of the wig.

Dr. Strawbridge told me about a surgical oncologist, Dr. Mary Hooks, who was with the Quillan School of Medicine at East Tennessee State University in Johnson City, Tennessee; she specialized exclusively in breast cancer patients. Dr. Strawbridge highly recommended her and I requested a referral. As expected, I was very pleased with the referral and got excellent care from Dr. Hooks.

Almost immediately after our discussion of my options at the first appointment with Dr. Hooks, I decided to have a reconstruction done. Prior to the surgery, she had me see Dr. Daniel Haynes, an excellent plastic surgeon, who was present at the initial surgery to do the first stage of the reconstruction. He had been unsure about a reconstruction because of my age—I was 65 at the time. Once he saw me, he said my skin was good enough to be able to handle the reconstruction.

In early March of 2007, once the surgical consultations were completed, I had a modified radical mastectomy of the left breast. The first three lymph nodes under my left arm showed the presence of cancer. Dr. Hooks removed them and then took out 6 more lymph nodes from under my arm; all of the additional nodes were negative for cancer. Dr. Haynes did the implant for the breast reconstruction at that initial surgery. The mass itself was fairly large, 2.5 to 3 centimeters in length. This meant I was essentially at an early stage 3 and was going to need radiation in addition to the chemotherapy.

Since I had to have a modified radical mastectomy (with the removal of the larger number of lymph nodes), I have a higher risk of developing lymphedema of the left arm. This is a generalized swelling of the arm, secondary to the poor drainage of lymph (intercellular fluid that is between the cells and drains back into the circulation through the lymphatic system) from the arm, because of the absence of the large number of lymph nodes. Fortunately, I have not had that complication. It did occur more frequently in women with breast cancer that I saw during my medical training. At that time all of the lymph nodes under the arm were taken out with the surgery and the entire breast and surrounding healthy tissue was taken as well. The surgery is much more limited now and is not as mutilating as those earlier surgeries were.

Prior to the chemotherapy I had some additional diagnostic tests, including a baseline MUGA scan, which measures the cardiac ejection fraction. This scan was done in radiology with radioactive isotopes, combined with a sample of my blood that was then injected back into my body for the scan.

This test provided a baseline to monitor for a possible cardiomyopathy, which is a weakening of the heart muscle, a relatively infrequent but serious side effect of the chemotherapy. When it occurs, it will cause heart failure that can be very serious and even result in death.

Dr. Hooks also put in an intravascular port under the skin on my right upper chest. It provides a port that can be used for IV infusions for the chemotherapy. It's connected to a tube that goes into the superior vena cava, the large vein for returning blood from the upper body to the heart. Its primary purpose is to provide IV access for the chemotherapy. It is also where blood is drawn to monitor for problems with the chemo, such as liver toxicity (damage) or decreased blood cells.

Dr. Hooks had sent the tumor to the pathology lab at the time of the mastectomy. This provided the final diagnosis of the type of cancer I had. It was also tested for estrogen sensitivity and for indicators of a genetic type of breast cancer, which is frequently one of the more aggressive of the breast cancers, and more likely to be transmitted genetically. These cancers tend to occur in younger women. Fortunately, I did not have that more aggressive type of tumor.

It was my choice to continue to work part-time, up until the initial surgery. I had been providing psychiatric services for the Children and Youth division at the Frontier Health - Bristol Regional

Counseling Center, and I could not have asked for a better work situation during such a difficult time. They allowed me to take six weeks off for the surgery and then return on a limited schedule for the duration of the chemotherapy, which took 5 to 6 months.

I did not have a really aggressive type of breast cancer and Dr. Prill gave me 4 treatments of IV Adriamycin and Cytoxin in combination, followed by 4 treatments of IV Taxotere for a total of 8 infusions given once every 3 weeks. The protocol was a standard one for my tumor type and was followed after I completed the radiation treatments, by 5 years of treatment with Femera (generic name is letrozole), one of the medications for estrogen suppression.

Dr. Prill used a mixture of additional medications before the infusions to minimize the side effects of the chemo. This included starting me on a high dose of steroids the day before the chemo and continuing through the day of the treatment and into the following day. Fortunately, I had reasonably good energy while I was on the steroids and would then crash the first day I was off of them. I had scheduled the treatments for Thursdays, so that I had time to recover from the treatment before starting back to work on Monday.

The treatments were given in a large room with anywhere from 4 to 11 other patients, who were also there for their treatments. There was a clean-up area in the bathroom off the infusion room in case anyone became violently ill during their treatment. The nurses were excellent and were particularly careful with me during the first treatment. I never saw anyone have a bad reaction to the treatments. I did experience a decrease in my white blood cells and was given injections to counteract that reaction to the chemo. My port became impossible to draw blood from after about 3 chemo treatments. This apparently is not that uncommon. Fortunately, it did not interfere with the primary purpose of the port, which was to provide IV access for the chemotherapy infusions.

The initial diagnostic work was done at the hospital in Abingdon, Virginia, which is where Dr. Strawbridge has her practice. The mastectomy and the initial reconstructive work were done at the Johnson City Medical Center in Johnson City, Tennessee. The remaining reconstructive surgeries were done at a small, community hospital in Erwin, Tennessee. It provided excellent care without the increased risk of MRSA that exists at the larger medical centers. MRSA is an antibiotic-resistant staph infection that can be very difficult to treat. Dr. Haynes does all his surgeries in that smaller setting, rather than in the larger medical settings, except when he does the initial breast implant at the time of a mastectomy.

The chemotherapy and later radiation were done at Wellmont-Bristol Regional Medical Center. Dr. John Fincher was the radiologist and again I received excellent care. My treatment plan was set up this way because I knew and had consulted at both the Abingdon and the Bristol hospitals. Having Dr. Hooks, with her very specialized knowledge and skills was the godsend that helped make local treatment possible. She brought in Dr. Haynes for the reconstruction and that completed the treatment team. Dr. Hooks moved on to Vanderbilt in Nashville about 4 years ago. I am still following up with all the other providers and have been fortunate to have had excellent care and follow-up available in my own community.

CHAPTER 2

Complications During Treatment

While there were no significant problems immediately following my initial surgery in March of 2007, I did have several complications as the additional treatments for my cancer continued. My suspicion is that this is not uncommon for patients undergoing treatment for cancers of all types.

The first issue surfaced in the aftermath of my first chemotherapy treatment. There were significant changes in my voice and I reported this to Dr. Prill immediately. There had not been any prior record of voice changes related to these treatments. However, on returning to work, my voice recognition software no longer recognized my post-treatment voice, which confirmed to me the changes were real.

I had been using the software for dictation of clinical notes for my patients at Frontier for several years and I knew right away there was no other reason for the problems with the software. I went ahead and contacted the woman, who had initially trained me on the software, to help me create a new profile that Dragon would recognize as me. We kept both versions of my profile on the computer so I could go back to the normal (for me) profile once the treatments were finished. Ultimately we had to do a third profile before the treatments were completed.

Once the chemotherapy was over, Dr. Haynes wanted to do a second stage of the breast reconstruction before I underwent the radiation treatments, since those treatments would be additionally traumatic to the remaining breast tissue. I thought that was a good idea and the surgery was scheduled.

I still had the voice changes and a cough, which had started around the same time as my voice changes. When the anesthesiologist heard about the cough he refused to do the anesthesia until I had had a pulmonary work-up. I knew I had no symptoms of lung disease and that the cough was a lesser problem going along with the voice changes. I kept telling him, "It's my larynx, not my lungs," but the anesthesiologist would not budge, so I had Kathy Sharp, the nurse practitioner in Dr. Prill's office, arrange a quick consult with an ENT (ear, nose, throat) doctor to check out my larynx. Dr. Alan Davis saw me within the week and I was happy with the referral. He had been the doctor who took care of my sons' ear infections when they were young and I had always had a good relationship with him through the years.

He numbed my nose and throat and then ran a tube down through my nose and into the larynx so we could both see my vocal cords on the computer monitor. They looked like a bright pink horseshoe, which is anything but normal. He said "You have GERD and you need to be on medication for that." GERD is short for Gastro-Esophageal Reflux Disorder and is a very common ailment. It occurs when the stomach contents, including stomach acid, backs up into the esophagus, causing heartburn and irritation to the back of the mouth and to the larynx or vocal cords. Dr. Davis gave me a prescription for Protonix®, to treat the reflux, and he spent some time on the phone, reassuring the anesthesiologist that there were no problems related to going ahead with the surgery as scheduled. As it turned out, my voice changes were not due to the chemo, but were a result of the high doses of steroids that were used to prevent the more severe side effects of the chemo.

The second surgery didn't result in any anesthesia problems. However, as I was waking up from the surgery, I developed a very itchy rash that looked like patches of poison ivy. Since I was still somewhat out of it from the drugs I had been given, I didn't say anything about it to the nurse. When Dr. Haynes came in a few minutes later, he ordered more steroids to stop the allergic reaction. We were both concerned that I might have to be admitted to the hospital overnight for observation. Luckily the rash was gone within an hour of the steroids and I was able to go home. However, I did see an allergist to try to figure out which of the drugs I was allergic to. The best guess was that it was the Keflex®, which was given because of my mitral valve prolapse (a relatively common congenital heart defect). I was able to get alternative drugs to all the medications that were given at that surgery for all the surgeries that followed, and had no more allergic reactions. At least not in connection with surgeries.

I did have one more allergic reaction — to the radioactive solution they administered for my last follow-up MUGA scan. I ended up having to go to the ER in Bristol to get treatment, because it came on about 36 hours after the scan. There were no other exposures besides that solution that weren't an ongoing part of my usual, daily routine. Fortunately the scan itself was normal (all three scans were normal) and I do not have to have that scan again. The test is important because, in some instances, the chemotherapy can cause a cardiomyopathy or severe weakening of the heart muscle. These scans will show that as a reduction in the heart's ejection fraction, meaning that the heart is weak and not pumping a normal amount of blood out to the body with each heart beat. This reaction occurred several months after the post-operative rash. These are the only two allergic reactions I have had during my lifetime.

Three weeks after I finished my radiation treatments I came down with the flu for the first time in over 30 years. I had a fever, severe muscle aches and capsulitis, which is an inflammation of the tissue around the breast implant. I had itching of the underlying breast tissue that lasted for about 36 hours and there was nothing I could do to make it better. Oddly enough, I did not have any of the nausea, vomiting, diarrhea, cold symptoms or chest congestion that almost everyone else had with the flu that year. Particularly considering my profession as a doctor, I've been blessed with good resistance to colds and flu and I saw this as merely a partial infection with the flu.

Fortunately, I was not seriously ill and after 24 hours of mild fever and muscle aches, the capsulitis was the only remaining problem. The itching went on for another 12 hours before it too went away. The capsulitis was likely an indicator of the sensitivity of the remaining tissue of the breast, due to the trauma from the treatments during the previous year.

After the third surgery, I developed significant inflammation, or severe irritation, of the skin over the breast, which was warm to the touch and very pink in color. It was definitely not normal and I called Dr. Haynes to let him know what was happening. He told me to go to the ER at Johnson City Medical Center and he met me there within the hour. It was on a weekend, but to my knowledge he always takes these kinds of calls himself, even on the weekends. He had already called in orders for blood work, mainly a CBC (complete blood count), and that had been drawn and sent to the lab before he arrived.

We were both concerned about the possibility of an infection of the breast. He examined the area and indicated that I would likely need to be admitted to the hospital for IV antibiotics. However, I had no fever or any other symptoms of infection. And besides, after spending two hours in the ER, I was getting very hungry. When my white blood count came back, it was 6000, which is normal for me. They sometimes say that doctors make the worst patients, and in this case maybe it's true; I decided to go home, as I did not think I had an infection. It was probably just some kind of non-specific inflammatory reaction of the skin to yet another surgery.

We talked the situation over at some length and he was clearly worried about sending me home. No doubt he would not have let me go had I not been a physician. With a promise that I would let him know and return immediately if anything got worse, he acquiesced. My first post-op check-up was in two days anyway. He told me that I should get some over-the-counter medication, Pepcid®, to take twice daily until I saw him again. There was apparently some research that indicated it was helpful with non-specific inflammation. So I took the Pepcid® and also used some coconut oil on the area. The inflammation was significantly improved by the time I saw him again two days later. He examined the breast very thoroughly and then grinned at me and said, "It looks like you made the right call."

Over the next two years I had two more surgeries for new implants. With each additional surgery, I had the inflammatory reaction with the capsulitis. It responded best to Motrin® every 8 hours, along with coconut oil. It became clear to me that I was not going to get a really normal looking breast without additional surgeries that involved moving skin and muscle in stages from my back, and moving them to the breast. Rather than go through all that, I decided against additional surgery, and determined to be satisfied with the existing outcome. It feels like I have a breast there and it looks OK under my clothing. Besides, I'm way past the age where I worry about looking like a model. I had that kind of figure in my twenties and thirties and it was fun. But I am in my seventies now and I can live with less.

Surviving Breast Cancer

CHAPTER 3

Self Care During Treatment

The good news was that radiation treatments were not as debilitating as chemotherapy. My energy remained reasonably good throughout the two months of treatments, from December, 2007 to January, 2008. Because of the holidays I had some extra days off between treatments, and this gave me more time to recover during the time I was undergoing the radiation. I had five treatments a week for eight weeks (4 during the holidays) and recovered my energy level much faster once the treatments were finished. As noted, I did get a limited case of the flu three weeks after radiation, which I believe was a result of the radiation's effect on my immune system. However, since I only had a low-grade fever and muscle aches without the usual gastrointestinal and upper respiratory symptoms, my immune system was still mostly protective against the full-blown symptoms of the flu.

However, that did not protect me from developing capsulitis around the breast implant with the same infection I described in the previous chapter. This would not be typical for the flu. I do believe that this was the most vulnerable part of my body in the aftermath of the radiation. The impact of the chemotherapy followed by the radiation treatments was the primary contributor to my having the flu for the first time in over 30 years. I had another infection with the flu the following year, during flu season. But aside from the capsulitis, which was part of that infection as well, there was no significant fever or fatigue, and muscle cramps were much milder with that last infection. As I continued to work with children and adolescents for the next six years, and have had no other episodes of flu or colds, I believe that my immune system is back to its normal effectiveness in warding off infections.

As I write this, it has been nine years since the initial diagnosis of breast cancer. Some credit must go to the changes in lifestyle I made prior to my diagnosis for preventing several of the worst side effects of chemotherapy, and to a lesser extent the radiation treatments. I also credit these and other changes with allowing me to remain in good health with no evidence of recurrence at this time. I have learned over the years to listen to my body's signals and to change my routine, if necessary, to accommodate my body's need for additional rest or other forms of care. I will do this when I am faced with increased symptoms of physical and/or emotional stress that I believe results in greater vulnerability to physical illnesses. For example, I battled migraine headaches for many years, but with the elimination of all caffeine and the dietary changes I made shortly before the diagnosis of cancer, I've remained completely free of migraines even during the treatments, and am migraine free to this day.

During the three years just prior to my diagnosis of cancer, I had fibromyalgia. In my opinion the fibromyalgia was a direct result of working in both inpatient and outpatient settings with the Department of Psychiatry at Bristol Regional Medical Center. We were three psychiatrists covering busy outpatient practices and two inpatient units after a fourth psychiatrist abruptly left the practice and returned to his native India. The result was that we were all on call every third night and every third weekend, and on call shifts were always busy. My sleep schedule was completely disrupted, and after three years I decided to retire at 62 rather than continuing to work those hours, which were so damaging to my physical wellbeing. To put it bluntly, I had no interest in retiring in a body bag.

The fibromyalgia symptoms gradually improved over the next several months, following this first retirement. With the dietary changes I made gradually over the next three years, and the improvement in my sleep once I was off call, the fibromyalgia had cleared completely before I started my cancer treatments. I later read about a study out of China that identified rotating shift work with its built-in sleep disruption as a factor in the increased incidence of breast cancer in women who worked those shifts for extended periods of time. So I now consider that brutal call schedule one of the causes of my own breast cancer.

The first change I made was about 12 years ago. After reading a report in one of my medical newsletters about the benefits of using hydrogen peroxide as a mouthwash, I made that switch and continue it to this day. I had always had a significant amount of plaque buildup along the gum line because I hated to floss and never developed the habit of doing so, in spite of several attempts to make it a part of my daily routine. There was always a lot of bleeding of the gums when I had my teeth cleaned every six months, but that was more acceptable to me than flossing on a regular basis.

My first cleaning after starting the hydrogen peroxide went much better and there was significantly less bleeding during that cleaning. This was about 5 months after starting the hydrogen peroxide. By the second cleaning there was very little bleeding and that has remained the case ever since. I gargle and then swish the peroxide around in my mouth and between my teeth for about 90 seconds.

When I then spit it out it is the consistency of thick whipped cream and my mouth feels very clean. I have had some unexpected benefits from this practice. First I have had bleaching of my teeth so that it looks like I am getting whitening treatments, which I guess I am on a daily basis. The peroxide costs about $0.59 a bottle and will usually last for 45 to 60 days. It only takes one half to one tablespoon of the peroxide to get the benefits. It is important to do the treatment immediately after brushing your teeth, as the bubbling up process of the peroxide does not work as well without the toothpaste. When you spit out the toothpaste you need to leave a small amount of the toothpaste in the back of your mouth to mix with the peroxide when you gargle with it. I had been doing this for several years before I got the cancer and I believe it protected me from the mouth sores that can be one of the more uncomfortable side effects of the chemotherapy.

I continued to do the fruit smoothies that I had started several weeks before I was diagnosed with the breast cancer. Shortly after starting the chemo I realized I was not having any of the gastrointestinal symptoms, such as nausea, vomiting or diarrhea that are common side effects. I immediately started using only organically grown fruits and also used almond and soy based milk substitutes in the smoothies. No matter what other fruits I used, I always added one to three bananas (depending on the size). I believe that these smoothies kept my gut healthy in the face of the damage that the chemo can do to that system. Chemo targets rapidly multiplying cells. The cells in the lining of the stomach and intestines are also rapidly multiplying, thus making them susceptible to the effects of the chemo, just like the rapidly multiplying cancer cells are. That is what makes the treatments effective in killing off the cancer cells.

Other cells in the body also suffer from these same effects. Another system is the blood cells, which are also more rapidly multiplying. I had a decrease in my white blood count and was given injections to stimulate the production of the blood cells and prevent anemia or a deficiency of the white cells that can make the immune system less effective in dealing with potentially infectious agents, bacteria or viruses, or any remaining cancer cells.

I was very careful to conserve my energy throughout the course of chemotherapy treatments, resting in the evenings and on the weekends for most of that time. I was able to be more active for several days before each new treatment and would try to get the necessary things done then, knowing that I wouldn't feel up to doing them once the next treatment began. One thing that was especially helpful in conserving my energy was the purchase of a shower stool and a Swedish shower head attached to a hose. These enabled me to bathe from a seated position. Showering from a standing position was often just too tiring.

I was able to keep up a limited schedule at work and I had good support from my colleagues there. Otherwise I did only the necessary basics and safeguarded my energy as much as possible. I had a lot of support from my son, who lived with me, and from the rest of my family and friends. All of them made it possible for me to get through the treatments much more easily than I had expected.

Being careful and taking good care of yourself can make a significant difference in how well or ill you can be during the course of traditional cancer treatments. I graduated medical school in 1966 and can tell you that cancer treatments have improved a lot since then. The surgery for my cancer was much more limited and the chemotherapy and radiation treatments were less toxic than what was available 40+ years ago. However, I also believe that utilizing some additional, nontraditional interventions can also improve your chances of survival long term and that is what I will discuss in more detail in the next chapter.

Surviving Breast Cancer

CHAPTER 4

Self Care Following Treatment

Let me make my position clear with respect to the issue of recurrence of cancer, no matter what type it is: I do not believe it is possible, in most instances, to ever remove every single cancer cell from the body, no matter how aggressive the treatments are. However it is possible to remove or destroy the vast majority of the cancer cells, and if the body's immune system is healthy enough it will take out or contain the remainder, and a complete cure will then be a possibility.

There are also a small number of cancers that will remit without treatment of any sort, but these are generally rare. For instance, when I was researching articles on the prognosis of thyroid cancer during my internship in 1967, there was a report of an elderly woman who was demented and was diagnosed with thyroid cancer. She was considered for an experimental treatment protocol, but she became one of the untreated controls. She resided in a nursing home and it was decided to send her back to the nursing home for supportive terminal care, given her dementia. Two years later, someone who was gathering data on the outcomes of patients and controls in the protocol study, contacted the nursing home to find out when she had died of her cancer. To their surprise, the nursing home staff reported that she was still alive and had no evidence of the cancer. A physician who examined her confirmed that she was free of cancer at that time. She is an example of an unusual instance of someone remitting without any treatment, either traditional or alternative.

I chose to take the recommended course of chemotherapy and radiation as this gave me a 60 to 70% chance of surviving at the end of 5 years. The chance of survival without the treatments was significantly lower, 35 to 40%. I did not have the inclination to try to research alternative treatments and try to make a reasonable decision in an area where I was not educated and where the different alternative treatments were not adequately researched. I did start reading some about cancer in general and the success or failures of a variety of treatments. With the help of Amazon.com, and its good suggestions of books related to my searches in this area, I happened upon a book by a physician, David Derry, MD titled *Breast Cancer and Iodine*. The book is a quick read and it gave me some very important information. He noted that the Japanese have the lowest incidence worldwide of all cancers, with the exception of stomach cancer. The stomach cancer appears to be secondary to the high use of nitrates in their diet.

The low incidence of all other cancers appears to be due to their high intake of iodine from eating large amounts of fish and seaweed daily, both excellent sources of iodine. The average person on the Japanese diet eats 8 to 10 mg of iodine daily. The iodine appears to be especially useful in the prevention of reproductive cancers in men and women. I learned about this shortly after my chemotherapy and I have been taking a 12.5 mg tablet of iodine daily since then. This was started almost eleven years ago now. The iodine is available through Amazon.com or iherb.com if you do not have a local source for that. I have always used the Iodoral™ brand, but that is not the only brand available through Amazon.

The iodine is necessary for the proper functioning of the thyroid gland and the thyroid will take all the iodine the body takes in if the iodine intake is insufficient. This leaves all the cells in the rest of the body with only the iodine available in the thyroid hormones, which is not optimal.

All cells in the body depend on the mitochondria, the part of the cell that provides energy for the cells' functioning. The mitochondria appear to be descended from ocean-dwelling single cell organisms that initially learned how to concentrate iodine in the cell, from the iodine that is in the ocean water in very dilute quantities. Iodine is one of the rare earth minerals, and these organisms developed a way to make it more available to their own cells by concentrating it about 3,000 times higher inside the cell from the concentration of iodine in the ocean water. This was clearly of significant survival value. Other cells that benefitted from the iodine concentrating ability then took in these organisms. These original organisms then became a part of these cells and eventually became part of multi-cell organisms and all the living things that have developed from them.

The iodine supplements provide the body with enough iodine to completely saturate the thyroid gland and have a lot left over for the other cells in the body. The reason that the iodine helps to prevent recurrence of cancer is that the connective tissue of the body, which essentially holds the rest of the body together as ligaments, tendons, connective tissue, etc., will tend to wall off and contain cancer cells within a connective tissue pocket. This prevents the cancer cells from spreading out into the rest of the body and they will eventually die off without causing any damage to the body as a whole. Japanese women have a high incidence of carcinoma in situ (cancer that has not invaded the connective tissue and spread beyond that pocket) and a very low incidence of actual breast cancer. This is what happens when the connective tissue is in good health. American women, on the other hand, have a low incidence of carcinoma in situ and a high incidence of breast cancer.

What I learned from my own experience with the iodine supplementation was that, after five to six months of taking the iodine, I had significantly improved mobility throughout my body. I was able to look back over my shoulder to check for other cars before changing lanes, something that had been more difficult as I got older. This had not improved when the rest of my fibromyalgia symptoms cleared and had actually been developing gradually even prior to the fibromyalgia. I now have good mobility overall, though I still don't move as fast as I did when I was younger.

I have continued to use the green smoothies for about nine or ten years now. I drink about a quart or more of a green smoothie and have done that since switching from the fruit smoothies that I had been drinking almost daily for about two years prior to the switch. In addition to providing some protection from recurrence of my breast cancer, it has also significantly increased my HDL cholesterol to 54. This was totally unexpected. Two years on a Nordic Track four or five times a week and some dietary changes for heart health had done nothing to improve my HDL cholesterol, which had remained in the mid-thirties for all of my adult life. Within the past few years I have added 1/2 of an organic lemon to each smoothie, peel and all, as there is some evidence from aromatherapy that lemon essential oil is helpful in the overall management of cancer. For the latest version of my green smoothie see the recipe in the back of the book.

I am currently losing weight, having been able to organize my diet more effectively since I retired from my consulting practice with the local mental health center at the end of August 2014. I have gradually lost 45 pounds, since starting in early September 2014 and I am continuing to lose weight on the green smoothies and one or two small meals a day. I have also started to experiment with coconut oil and other coconut products in place of some of dairy products and avoid wheat and grain products that are loaded with pesticides and/or are genetically modified. I am staying with organic foods as much as possible, as I believe the non-organic and GMO foods are a risk factor for cancer as well as other health problems, including diabetes, heart disease and obesity. I am feeling better generally since I have had the time to take better care of myself and am convinced this will continue to help reduce my risk of a cancer recurrence.

The last thing that I have added to my prevention strategy is a Native American herbal supplement that I learned about through one of my coworkers at the mental health center. She and her husband had gotten a puppy several years ago and the puppy had a large vascular tumor in his throat, which was growing very fast and making it almost impossible for him to swallow and take in his food. Their vet had told them to keep the dog as comfortable as possible until he reached the point when he needed to be put down. A friend of hers told her about the herbal supplement, Ojibwa Herbal Extract, 450 mg capsules. They saw no reason not to try it. They opened the capsule and dumped the powder into the puppy's food twice a day. Within a few weeks the tumor was decreasing in size and it continued to become smaller until it was completely gone by the time he was one year old. He is now over 5 years old and is a healthy and normally active dog. The day she told me about that, I looked the supplement up on Amazon and ordered my first supply. I have been taking it for five to six years now and I will continue to use it for the rest of my life, just like the iodine and the smoothies.

The only other medication that I take regularly is Armor® thyroid 120 mg daily for my hypothyroidism, which I have had for over 20 years. I had initially been on Synthroid® 100 mcg daily for about eight or nine years. I changed to a combination of Synthroid® and Cytomel®, which gave me coverage with both T3 and T4. These are the most common thyroid hormones, but they are not the only ones the thyroid produces. The dose was increased to 125 mcg daily when I was on the combination. After I read the information in the book by Dr. Derry, *Breast Cancer and Iodine*, and his recommendation to switch to the natural thyroid hormone I started taking the Armor® thyroid and feel better on that. It gives me all the thyroid hormones, not just T3 and T4. And my overall dosage has decreased to its original level. I've been on the Armor® thyroid for ten or eleven years now and will continue to be on it for the rest of my life.

Plenty of information circulates on the Internet regarding cancer treatments and the pros and cons of using either the traditional medical treatments or the alternative treatments. I do not believe that this should be an either/or decision. I am very satisfied with the treatment I have received from Drs. Strawbridge, Hooks, Haynes, Prill, Sharp and Fincher in the traditional treatments for the cancer. I am also glad I am maintaining my health with the treatments noted above, that fall outside of traditional medicine.

Every individual who receives a diagnosis of cancer has a right to make his or her own decisions regarding the treatments that are most acceptable. Using a combination of treatments as I have done would seem to be a reasonable approach, especially if improving one's overall health status and quality of life is the focus of those decisions. There are no absolute right or wrong decisions here, only what will most effectively provide for the quality of life that you wish to strive for.

There is only one other recommendation I have, which is not health related. This is for women who have had a single mastectomy or double mastectomies and are experiencing uneven contours in the reconstructed breast(s). Personally, I had gone without wearing a bra for most of 8 years after the mastectomy, because I was unable to find a bra that would work with both breasts. I had gained weight during and after the cancer treatments, and my breasts were significantly different in size. I had tried the breast prosthesis that was weighted to simulate the weight of a normal breast, but it was just too uncomfortable and irritating to my skin over the implant and I stopped wearing it within two days.

Once I lost the weight, I could fit into an XL-size sports bra. The ones I ordered have worked very well. They contain a removable cup that can be used to modify the contours of the breast and while my left breast is still somewhat smaller than my right, they appear to be roughly the same size when I wear the bra under clothes, even tee shirts. I am still losing weight, and I expect the breasts will be close to the same size with another 10 to 15 pound-weight loss. The bras are very comfortable and I have been very pleased with them. I ordered mine online through Jockey.com. I have not seen any other bras that have a removable cup and it is this feature that gives them the flexibility to add or remove small contoured padding and which smoothe out irregular contours for the reconstructed breast that remains after all the surgeries.

Every patient with breast cancer faces a difficult time and difficult decisions. I have given my story as one example of how I, with the advantage of a physician's knowledge, went through the process of putting together a treatment plan for my breast cancer. With good referrals I was able to put together the treatment team that provided the appropriate care for me. Your decisions, of course, may be quite different.

Most women who are diagnosed with breast cancer do not have the advantage that I did, because they have not been involved in the healthcare industry. I do hope that this account will be useful to those women who are faced with this diagnosis and that it will give them the confidence to take an active part in developing their own treatment plans. Cancer treatments are improving all the time and good medical care is available with the traditional cancer treatments for breast cancer. Also, eliminating some of the lifestyle issues that put you more at risk, along with prayers and support from friends and family, will give you the best chance of a good outcome with this illness.

CHAPTER 5

Philip's Story

It was 1971 when I met Philip Liverman, toward the end of my year as chief resident in psychiatry at the University of Virginia Hospital. He had just started dating my close friend, Joan Hulley. She was a second-year resident in psychiatry and he was a third year medical student on psychiatry. Although he was five years younger than Joan, and they had not been dating for very long — I could see how much she was enjoying her time with him.

As their relationship was beginning, I was going to Washington DC twice a week from Charlottesville, for my training analysis at the Washington Psychoanalytic Institute. My plan was to move to the DC area as soon as I completed my last residency year. Philip's family lived in Georgetown and he needed a ride home as he didn't have a car at that time. Joan asked if I could give him a ride up and of course I did. As I was still learning my way around Washington, I knew he could direct me to his home and also back to Connecticut Avenue to make my appointment with my analyst.

Not knowing him well yet, I wasn't sure what to expect on the ride up. However, we talked non-stop all the way to DC and surprisingly it was one of the more enjoyable encounters I have had under similar circumstances. We both learned about each other in a number of ways, discussing childhood experiences and challenges, as well as medical training and interests. It made the trip fun and the time passed quickly.

About halfway to DC, there was a brief lull in the conversation and then he said, "I'm going to marry her." Just like that. No hesitation. No qualifying of his intentions. Just the simple statement. I was very impressed by his commitment and by his confidence in pursuing the relationship. When telling Joan about this later, she smiled and said that dating him was very different for her. He had grown up in France and was very European in his attitude toward women. She said dating him made her realize how tentative most American relationships could be. As it turned out, they did marry and I was the maid of honor at the wedding. Since we lived in different locations, I didn't see much of them over the next several years but did maintain some contact with Joan.

In 1982 I got a call from her — Philip had cancer and they were in the process of having it diagnosed. He had a very rare tumor on one of the joints on his left ring finger. He had it biopsied and the specimen was sent to the top eight cancer centers in the country. Seven of the eight diagnosed it as a clear cell sarcoma. The eighth center, Memorial Sloan Kettering, diagnosed it as an amelanotic melanoma. Both tumor types diagnosed are extremely aggressive cancers and would require aggressive, although quite different, chemotherapy treatments. Because of the agreement of the seven centers that it was a clear cell sarcoma, he underwent the treatment for that with a radical amputation of the finger and part of his hand, followed by the specified chemotherapy. The side effects of the chemo were grueling, but he had been confident that he had a good chance at a cure with the treatment and was determined to see the full course through. Eighteen months after the therapy, he developed additional cancer in the lymph nodes under his left arm. Tragically, it became clear that the lone Memorial Sloan Kettering diagnosis had been correct. He had amelanotic melanoma, not clear cell sarcoma. He underwent additional treatment with the appropriate drugs, but it was too little too late and he ultimately died of his cancer.

They moved back to DC to live with his mother in Georgetown for the final stages of his illness. I was able to spend some time with Joan, and saw him once more toward the end of his illness — I was very sad for both of them and also for their two young children. Joan and Philip had been very fortunate to have one of the good marriages. It was tragic for them that he lost his life so early in their lives together.

When I think of Philip, I always remember that trip when I took him to DC, and in his honor, I have contributed to Memorial Sloan Kettering for a number of years. Why MSK was the only cancer center that got his diagnosis right, I will probably never know. I don't know if anyone checked with them to determine how they made the diagnosis they did. It is very sad that he received treatment for the wrong cancer and didn't survive the error. He was an excellent physician and nephrologist and it was such a loss that he died so early in his professional life. He is still remembered at the medical school with the annual Liverman Lecture in Nephrology. He was a loving husband and father, and his death was very hard for Joan and his children. Supporting cancer research and treatment at MSK is for me a fitting way to remember him, and honor his family's loss.

If you would like to join me, donations may be made online at: http://mskcc.convio.net/goto/SurvivingBreastCancer

If you prefer, donations may also be sent by mail, in memory of Philip Liverman, c/o MSK Foundation, 1275 York Aveune, New York, NY 10065. For further information, call 800-585-4118.

RESOURCES

1. *Breast Cancer and Iodine: How to Prevent and How to Survive Breast Cancer* by David Derry, MD - available through Amazon.com or other retail bookstores.

2. Iodoral Iodine Supplement, 12.5 mg tablet once daily. This brand comes in more than one strength so make sure to get this dose which is a slightly higher daily dose than the average Japanese dietary intake of 8 to 10 mg daily through fish and seaweed. If you have had an allergic reaction to iodine or iodine-containing products you will probably not be able to use this intervention. This brand of the iodine supplement is available through Amazon.com and usually costs between $30 and $40 per bottle of 180 tablets. If the price on Amazon is significantly higher than that, the same brand can probably be found cheaper on iherb.com in their minerals section.

3. Ojibwa Herbal Supplement 450 mg capsules, taken three times a day. It is a supplement that was developed and used by a native American tribe residing in Canada. They had used it with good benefit for many generations prior to allowing it to be released on the open market. I think the only brand for this supplement is NOW. It is available through Amazon.com and iherb.com. Amazon's prices are slightly better, but their source

for the Iodoral Iodine supplement has had prices up to $130/ bottle at one point 2 years ago and iherb.com did not have a similar price increase on the Iodoral at that time. Also iherb.com has a massive list of herbal supplements through NOW (723) as well as vitamins and other foods, such as protein powders for smoothies. It is worth checking out for anything that you want to try as a result of your own research.

4. I have used Armour Thyroid Hormone for the past 9 to 10 years in place of Synthroid and Cytomel, which are the pharmaceutically developed synthetic thyroid hormones. I believe this was a recommendation from Dr. Derry's book, but may also have come from one of the other books I read at the time. I have been on thyroid hormones for over 25 years and I have gotten better results with the natural Armour Thyroid Hormone which is derived from pig thyroid glands. Armour used to be less expensive than the synthetics. The price has gone up in the past five years and I don't know how it compares with the prices of the synthetics at this time.

5. I regularly have about a quart or more of a green smoothie in about three or four servings over the course of the day. I have included my recipe as another part of this book following the resources section. There is a lot of information available at the website www.greensmoothiegirl.com, including books available

through her shop. She also has a link to a site for a Blendtec blender at a discounted price. It is a very heavy duty blender and I have had mine for eight years without any problems. I would advise buying the larger blender jar which will hold 44 ounces because of the amount of smoothie you will want to make for the daily amount. I have only used the blender for smoothies and it does have a dedicated smoothie button which makes things simpler.

6. I purchased a colloidal silver generator which makes nanoparticles of silver suspended in a solution of distilled water. This is very helpful for external treatments for scrapes or small burns to the skin and helps to form a good scab to protect the injured area until it can heal. At that point the scab will then just fall off. It can also be taken internally for relief of pain. The dose I use is 30 to 60 ml (2 to 4 Tbsp) and the small cups that come with cold and cough liquid remedies give a good measure of 30 ml. This works best if combined with an anti-inflammatory such as ibuprofen or naproxen. I take 60 ml with 250 mg of naproxen once or twice daily if I am having pain and the combination works better than either one alone. I purchased the equipment for making the silver solution through Steve Barwick of www.thesilveredge.com. The silver solution can also help heal skin infections and can be used as

a sterilizing agent in cleaning countertops and other surfaces to prevent spread of disease. I have had no side effects to the colloidal silver. However, if colloidal silver is used in very high doses over an extended period of time it can turn your skin blue. The issues with finding the appropriate dose to avoid this are on the web site.

7. I also recently began to use a product called EASE which is a spray that can be used to provide a readily absorbed form of magnesium, a mineral that is essential to the overall health of the body, but one which most of us are deficient in. It absorbs easily through the skin and, when sprayed or rubbed on the skin, will be dry within 5 to 10 minutes. It helps with pain and can provide relief within a few minutes to areas of pain in the body. It can also be used over the body to provide for more magnesium generally to your body, even in the absence of pain issues. It is especially helpful with musculoskeletal pain and joint pain. It apparently will aid with improved calcification to injured areas, such as broken bones that are healing, though you will not be able to use it directly if the break is casted. You can use it directly for broken ribs or toes which are never casted or bound any more, as they will heal without the cast. It is helpful in the treatment of chronic pain and may reduce the need for pain medications. It is available through www.

easemagnesium.com. This is a Canadian company and some bank debit cards will not work for orders if the bank has a ban on any charges from outside the United States. The bank will usually approve a single purchase with confirmation from you that you have placed the order. They will usually not do automatic monthly orders if you choose to do that, which I have done. I had to use a different bank to get that set up. The company is Activation Products and can be reached by phone at (866) 271-7595. Their customer service has been very good in my experience.

MY BASIC GREEN SMOOTHIE RECIPE

Ingredients

1 box of organic baby lettuce or spinach – 4 to 5 oz.

1 500 ml container of coconut water

1 12 to 16 oz. bag of frozen fruit, thawed

1 organic kiwi – cut into small chunks (peel if not organic)

2 to 3 bananas – sliced into medium chunks

Most of these ingredients can be found at your local grocery (I find them at Food City or Kroger) or on Amazon.com

Directions

Place organic lettuce into a heavy-duty blender. Add the organic coconut water to the lettuce and blend for 25 seconds on puree or the smoothie setting, if your blender has that. Next, add the bagged fruit to the blender contents and blend for another 25 seconds.

Finally, add kiwi and bananas and blend for another 25 seconds. Pour into glasses and/or containers for later use. This recipe will make 1 to 1 1/2 quarts and will keep for 1 to 2 days in the refrigerator. Enjoy!

AFTERWORD

Congratulations on finishing this book. I hope it has been helpful. I have written it specifically for women who have been recently diagnosed with breast cancer and who are trying to cope with that new reality in their lives. They are also having to take in a lot of new information, especially if they do not have a medical background. And they are trying to begin to make decisions regarding their own treatments. I can remember what that was like when I was coming to terms with my own diagnosis of this difficult and scary disease. This is one of several books I have written; for this one, I've deliberately kept it as short and informative as possible, so the necessary information would be available within a short read. Certainly, I do not claim to have all the answers. Each of us is a unique individual and every woman will have her own story with her illness and treatments. I hope this will allow others to approach their journey through this process with acceptance and hope for their own recovery.

ABOUT THE AUTHOR

Dr. Linda R. Thompson has been a practicing physician in the area of psychiatry since 1966, when she graduated from the University of Virginia School of Medicine. A true pioneer at the time, she was one of only three women in her med school class. She went on to complete a rotating internship at the State University of Iowa Hospital in 1967, and she returned to the University of Virginia Hospital for her residency in psychiatry from 1967-1971.

She graduated in 1983 from an extensive ten-year psychoanalytic training program at the Washington Psychoanalytic Institute, while also running an active private practice in the Washington DC area. Returning to her native East Tennessee, she maintained a general psychiatric practice serving Northeast Tennessee and Southwest

Virginia from 1984 through 2014. Today, she continues to maintain a part-time general psychiatric and psychotherapy practice and devotes much of her time to writing.

This updated version of *Surviving Breast Cancer* joins her other books, including *Return to Asylums*, and *Old School Medicine*. She is currently researching and writing about Attention Deficit Hyperactivity Disorder (ADHD) and how this condition evolved.

www.ingramcontent.com/pod-product-compliance
Lightning Source LLC
Chambersburg PA
CBHW022132280326
41933CB00007B/656